CLIENT BOOK
FOR HAIR STYLISTS

____

____

____

Copyright© Write On Purpose Journals 2020

INDEX

NAME	PAGE

NAME

PAGE

NAME

PAGE

CLIENT

DATE | TIME

PHONE | EMAIL

SERVICE | DURATION

SUPPLIES

NOTES

CLIENT

DATE | TIME

PHONE | EMAIL

SERVICE | DURATION

SUPPLIES

NOTES

CLIENT

DATE | TIME

PHONE | EMAIL

SERVICE | DURATION

SUPPLIES

NOTES

CLIENT

DATE | TIME

PHONE | EMAIL

SERVICE | DURATION

SUPPLIES

NOTES

CLIENT

DATE	TIME
PHONE	EMAIL
SERVICE	DURATION

SUPPLIES

NOTES

CLIENT

DATE	TIME
PHONE	EMAIL
SERVICE	DURATION

SUPPLIES

NOTES

CLIENT

DATE	TIME
PHONE	EMAIL
SERVICE	DURATION

SUPPLIES

NOTES

CLIENT

DATE	TIME
PHONE	EMAIL
SERVICE	DURATION

SUPPLIES

NOTES

CLIENT

DATE	TIME
PHONE	EMAIL
SERVICE	DURATION

SUPPLIES

NOTES

CLIENT

DATE	TIME
PHONE	EMAIL
SERVICE	DURATION

SUPPLIES

NOTES

CLIENT

DATE | TIME

PHONE | EMAIL

SERVICE | DURATION

SUPPLIES

NOTES

CLIENT

DATE | TIME

PHONE | EMAIL

SERVICE | DURATION

SUPPLIES

NOTES

CLIENT

DATE	TIME
PHONE	EMAIL
SERVICE	DURATION

SUPPLIES

NOTES

CLIENT

DATE	TIME
PHONE	EMAIL
SERVICE	DURATION

SUPPLIES

NOTES

CLIENT

DATE	TIME
PHONE	EMAIL
SERVICE	DURATION

SUPPLIES

NOTES

CLIENT

DATE	TIME
PHONE	EMAIL
SERVICE	DURATION

SUPPLIES

NOTES

CLIENT

DATE | TIME

PHONE | EMAIL

SERVICE | DURATION

SUPPLIES

NOTES

CLIENT

DATE | TIME

PHONE | EMAIL

SERVICE | DURATION

SUPPLIES

NOTES

CLIENT

DATE	TIME
PHONE	EMAIL
SERVICE	DURATION

SUPPLIES

NOTES

CLIENT

DATE	TIME
PHONE	EMAIL
SERVICE	DURATION

SUPPLIES

NOTES

CLIENT

DATE	TIME
PHONE	EMAIL
SERVICE	DURATION

SUPPLIES

NOTES

CLIENT

DATE	TIME
PHONE	EMAIL
SERVICE	DURATION

SUPPLIES

NOTES

CLIENT

DATE	TIME
PHONE	EMAIL
SERVICE	DURATION

SUPPLIES

NOTES

CLIENT

DATE	TIME
PHONE	EMAIL
SERVICE	DURATION

SUPPLIES

NOTES

CLIENT

DATE	TIME
PHONE	EMAIL
SERVICE	DURATION

SUPPLIES

NOTES

CLIENT

DATE	TIME
PHONE	EMAIL
SERVICE	DURATION

SUPPLIES

NOTES

CLIENT

DATE	TIME
PHONE	EMAIL
SERVICE	DURATION

SUPPLIES

NOTES

CLIENT

DATE	TIME
PHONE	EMAIL
SERVICE	DURATION

SUPPLIES

NOTES

CLIENT

DATE | TIME

PHONE | EMAIL

SERVICE | DURATION

SUPPLIES

NOTES

CLIENT

DATE | TIME

PHONE | EMAIL

SERVICE | DURATION

SUPPLIES

NOTES

CLIENT

DATE	TIME
PHONE	EMAIL
SERVICE	DURATION

SUPPLIES

NOTES

CLIENT

DATE	TIME
PHONE	EMAIL
SERVICE	DURATION

SUPPLIES

NOTES

CLIENT

DATE	TIME
PHONE	EMAIL
SERVICE	DURATION

SUPPLIES

NOTES

CLIENT

DATE	TIME
PHONE	EMAIL
SERVICE	DURATION

SUPPLIES

NOTES

CLIENT

DATE	TIME
PHONE	EMAIL
SERVICE	DURATION

SUPPLIES

NOTES

CLIENT

DATE	TIME
PHONE	EMAIL
SERVICE	DURATION

SUPPLIES

NOTES

CLIENT

DATE	TIME
PHONE	EMAIL
SERVICE	DURATION

SUPPLIES

NOTES

CLIENT

DATE	TIME
PHONE	EMAIL
SERVICE	DURATION

SUPPLIES

NOTES

CLIENT

DATE	TIME
PHONE	EMAIL
SERVICE	DURATION

SUPPLIES

NOTES

CLIENT

DATE	TIME
PHONE	EMAIL
SERVICE	DURATION

SUPPLIES

NOTES

CLIENT

DATE	TIME
PHONE	EMAIL
SERVICE	DURATION

SUPPLIES

NOTES

CLIENT

DATE	TIME
PHONE	EMAIL
SERVICE	DURATION

SUPPLIES

NOTES

CLIENT

DATE	TIME
PHONE	EMAIL
SERVICE	DURATION

SUPPLIES

NOTES

CLIENT

DATE	TIME
PHONE	EMAIL
SERVICE	DURATION

SUPPLIES

NOTES

CLIENT

DATE	TIME
PHONE	EMAIL
SERVICE	DURATION

SUPPLIES

NOTES

CLIENT

DATE	TIME
PHONE	EMAIL
SERVICE	DURATION

SUPPLIES

NOTES

CLIENT

DATE	TIME
PHONE	EMAIL
SERVICE	DURATION

SUPPLIES

NOTES

CLIENT

DATE	TIME
PHONE	EMAIL
SERVICE	DURATION

SUPPLIES

NOTES

CLIENT

DATE	TIME
PHONE	EMAIL
SERVICE	DURATION

SUPPLIES

NOTES

CLIENT

DATE	TIME
PHONE	EMAIL
SERVICE	DURATION

SUPPLIES

NOTES

CLIENT

DATE | TIME

PHONE | EMAIL

SERVICE | DURATION

SUPPLIES

NOTES

CLIENT

DATE | TIME

PHONE | EMAIL

SERVICE | DURATION

SUPPLIES

NOTES

CLIENT

DATE | TIME

PHONE | EMAIL

SERVICE | DURATION

SUPPLIES

NOTES

CLIENT

DATE | TIME

PHONE | EMAIL

SERVICE | DURATION

SUPPLIES

NOTES

CLIENT

DATE	TIME
PHONE	EMAIL
SERVICE	DURATION

SUPPLIES

NOTES

CLIENT

DATE	TIME
PHONE	EMAIL
SERVICE	DURATION

SUPPLIES

NOTES

CLIENT

DATE	TIME
PHONE	EMAIL
SERVICE	DURATION

SUPPLIES

NOTES

CLIENT

DATE	TIME
PHONE	EMAIL
SERVICE	DURATION

SUPPLIES

NOTES

CLIENT

DATE	TIME
PHONE	EMAIL
SERVICE	DURATION

SUPPLIES

NOTES

CLIENT

DATE	TIME
PHONE	EMAIL
SERVICE	DURATION

SUPPLIES

NOTES

CLIENT

DATE	TIME
PHONE	EMAIL
SERVICE	DURATION

SUPPLIES

NOTES

CLIENT

DATE	TIME
PHONE	EMAIL
SERVICE	DURATION

SUPPLIES

NOTES

CLIENT

DATE	TIME
PHONE	EMAIL
SERVICE	DURATION

SUPPLIES

NOTES

CLIENT

DATE	TIME
PHONE	EMAIL
SERVICE	DURATION

SUPPLIES

NOTES

CLIENT

DATE	TIME
PHONE	EMAIL
SERVICE	DURATION

SUPPLIES

NOTES

CLIENT

DATE	TIME
PHONE	EMAIL
SERVICE	DURATION

SUPPLIES

NOTES

CLIENT

DATE	TIME
PHONE	EMAIL
SERVICE	DURATION

SUPPLIES

NOTES

CLIENT

DATE	TIME
PHONE	EMAIL
SERVICE	DURATION

SUPPLIES

NOTES

CLIENT

DATE	TIME
PHONE	EMAIL
SERVICE	DURATION

SUPPLIES

NOTES

CLIENT

DATE	TIME
PHONE	EMAIL
SERVICE	DURATION

SUPPLIES

NOTES

CLIENT

DATE | TIME

PHONE | EMAIL

SERVICE | DURATION

SUPPLIES

NOTES

CLIENT

DATE | TIME

PHONE | EMAIL

SERVICE | DURATION

SUPPLIES

NOTES

CLIENT

DATE	TIME
PHONE	EMAIL
SERVICE	DURATION

SUPPLIES

NOTES

CLIENT

DATE	TIME
PHONE	EMAIL
SERVICE	DURATION

SUPPLIES

NOTES

CLIENT

DATE | TIME

PHONE | EMAIL

SERVICE | DURATION

SUPPLIES

NOTES

CLIENT

DATE | TIME

PHONE | EMAIL

SERVICE | DURATION

SUPPLIES

NOTES

CLIENT

DATE	TIME
PHONE	EMAIL
SERVICE	DURATION

SUPPLIES

NOTES

CLIENT

DATE	TIME
PHONE	EMAIL
SERVICE	DURATION

SUPPLIES

NOTES

CLIENT

DATE	TIME
PHONE	EMAIL
SERVICE	DURATION

SUPPLIES

NOTES

CLIENT

DATE	TIME
PHONE	EMAIL
SERVICE	DURATION

SUPPLIES

NOTES

CLIENT

DATE	TIME
PHONE	EMAIL
SERVICE	DURATION

SUPPLIES

NOTES

CLIENT

DATE	TIME
PHONE	EMAIL
SERVICE	DURATION

SUPPLIES

NOTES

CLIENT

DATE	TIME
PHONE	EMAIL
SERVICE	DURATION

SUPPLIES

NOTES

CLIENT

DATE	TIME
PHONE	EMAIL
SERVICE	DURATION

SUPPLIES

NOTES

CLIENT

DATE	TIME
PHONE	EMAIL
SERVICE	DURATION

SUPPLIES

NOTES

CLIENT

DATE	TIME
PHONE	EMAIL
SERVICE	DURATION

SUPPLIES

NOTES

CLIENT

DATE	TIME
PHONE	EMAIL
SERVICE	DURATION

SUPPLIES

NOTES

CLIENT

DATE	TIME
PHONE	EMAIL
SERVICE	DURATION

SUPPLIES

NOTES

CLIENT

DATE | TIME

PHONE | EMAIL

SERVICE | DURATION

SUPPLIES

NOTES

CLIENT

DATE | TIME

PHONE | EMAIL

SERVICE | DURATION

SUPPLIES

NOTES

CLIENT

DATE	TIME
PHONE	EMAIL
SERVICE	DURATION

SUPPLIES

NOTES

CLIENT

DATE	TIME
PHONE	EMAIL
SERVICE	DURATION

SUPPLIES

NOTES

CLIENT

DATE	TIME
PHONE	EMAIL
SERVICE	DURATION

SUPPLIES

NOTES

CLIENT

DATE	TIME
PHONE	EMAIL
SERVICE	DURATION

SUPPLIES

NOTES

CLIENT

DATE	TIME
PHONE	EMAIL
SERVICE	DURATION

SUPPLIES

NOTES

CLIENT

DATE	TIME
PHONE	EMAIL
SERVICE	DURATION

SUPPLIES

NOTES

CLIENT

DATE	TIME
PHONE	EMAIL
SERVICE	DURATION

SUPPLIES

NOTES

CLIENT

DATE	TIME
PHONE	EMAIL
SERVICE	DURATION

SUPPLIES

NOTES

CLIENT

DATE	TIME
PHONE	EMAIL
SERVICE	DURATION

SUPPLIES

NOTES

CLIENT

DATE	TIME
PHONE	EMAIL
SERVICE	DURATION

SUPPLIES

NOTES

CLIENT

DATE	TIME
PHONE	EMAIL
SERVICE	DURATION

SUPPLIES

NOTES

CLIENT

DATE	TIME
PHONE	EMAIL
SERVICE	DURATION

SUPPLIES

NOTES

CLIENT

DATE	TIME
PHONE	EMAIL
SERVICE	DURATION

SUPPLIES

NOTES

CLIENT

DATE	TIME
PHONE	EMAIL
SERVICE	DURATION

SUPPLIES

NOTES

CLIENT

DATE	TIME
PHONE	EMAIL
SERVICE	DURATION

SUPPLIES

NOTES

CLIENT

DATE	TIME
PHONE	EMAIL
SERVICE	DURATION

SUPPLIES

NOTES

CLIENT

DATE	TIME
PHONE	EMAIL
SERVICE	DURATION

SUPPLIES

NOTES

CLIENT

DATE	TIME
PHONE	EMAIL
SERVICE	DURATION

SUPPLIES

NOTES

CLIENT

DATE	TIME
PHONE	EMAIL
SERVICE	DURATION

SUPPLIES

NOTES

CLIENT

DATE	TIME
PHONE	EMAIL
SERVICE	DURATION

SUPPLIES

NOTES

CLIENT

DATE | TIME

PHONE | EMAIL

SERVICE | DURATION

SUPPLIES

NOTES

CLIENT

DATE | TIME

PHONE | EMAIL

SERVICE | DURATION

SUPPLIES

NOTES

CLIENT

DATE	TIME
PHONE	EMAIL
SERVICE	DURATION

SUPPLIES

NOTES

CLIENT

DATE	TIME
PHONE	EMAIL
SERVICE	DURATION

SUPPLIES

NOTES

CLIENT

DATE	TIME
PHONE	EMAIL
SERVICE	DURATION

SUPPLIES

NOTES

CLIENT

DATE	TIME
PHONE	EMAIL
SERVICE	DURATION

SUPPLIES

NOTES

CLIENT

DATE	TIME
PHONE	EMAIL
SERVICE	DURATION

SUPPLIES

NOTES

CLIENT

DATE	TIME
PHONE	EMAIL
SERVICE	DURATION

SUPPLIES

NOTES

CLIENT

DATE	TIME
PHONE	EMAIL
SERVICE	DURATION

SUPPLIES

NOTES

CLIENT

DATE	TIME
PHONE	EMAIL
SERVICE	DURATION

SUPPLIES

NOTES

CLIENT

DATE	TIME
PHONE	EMAIL
SERVICE	DURATION

SUPPLIES

NOTES

CLIENT

DATE	TIME
PHONE	EMAIL
SERVICE	DURATION

SUPPLIES

NOTES

CLIENT

DATE	TIME
PHONE	EMAIL
SERVICE	DURATION

SUPPLIES

NOTES

CLIENT

DATE	TIME
PHONE	EMAIL
SERVICE	DURATION

SUPPLIES

NOTES

CLIENT

DATE	TIME
PHONE	EMAIL
SERVICE	DURATION

SUPPLIES

NOTES

CLIENT

DATE	TIME
PHONE	EMAIL
SERVICE	DURATION

SUPPLIES

NOTES

CLIENT

DATE	TIME
PHONE	EMAIL
SERVICE	DURATION

SUPPLIES

NOTES

CLIENT

DATE	TIME
PHONE	EMAIL
SERVICE	DURATION

SUPPLIES

NOTES

CLIENT

DATE	TIME
PHONE	EMAIL
SERVICE	DURATION

SUPPLIES

NOTES

CLIENT

DATE	TIME
PHONE	EMAIL
SERVICE	DURATION

SUPPLIES

NOTES

CLIENT

DATE	TIME
PHONE	EMAIL
SERVICE	DURATION

SUPPLIES

NOTES

CLIENT

DATE	TIME
PHONE	EMAIL
SERVICE	DURATION

SUPPLIES

NOTES

CLIENT

DATE	TIME
PHONE	EMAIL
SERVICE	DURATION

SUPPLIES

NOTES

CLIENT

DATE	TIME
PHONE	EMAIL
SERVICE	DURATION

SUPPLIES

NOTES

CLIENT

DATE	TIME
PHONE	EMAIL
SERVICE	DURATION

SUPPLIES

NOTES

CLIENT

DATE	TIME
PHONE	EMAIL
SERVICE	DURATION

SUPPLIES

NOTES

CLIENT

DATE	TIME
PHONE	EMAIL
SERVICE	DURATION

SUPPLIES

NOTES

CLIENT

DATE	TIME
PHONE	EMAIL
SERVICE	DURATION

SUPPLIES

NOTES

CLIENT

DATE	TIME
PHONE	EMAIL
SERVICE	DURATION

SUPPLIES

NOTES

CLIENT

DATE	TIME
PHONE	EMAIL
SERVICE	DURATION

SUPPLIES

NOTES

CLIENT

DATE	TIME
PHONE	EMAIL
SERVICE	DURATION

SUPPLIES

NOTES

CLIENT

DATE	TIME
PHONE	EMAIL
SERVICE	DURATION

SUPPLIES

NOTES

CLIENT

DATE	TIME
PHONE	EMAIL
SERVICE	DURATION

SUPPLIES

NOTES

CLIENT

DATE	TIME
PHONE	EMAIL
SERVICE	DURATION

SUPPLIES

NOTES

CLIENT

DATE	TIME
PHONE	EMAIL
SERVICE	DURATION

SUPPLIES

NOTES

CLIENT

DATE	TIME
PHONE	EMAIL
SERVICE	DURATION

SUPPLIES

NOTES

CLIENT

DATE	TIME
PHONE	EMAIL
SERVICE	DURATION

SUPPLIES

NOTES

CLIENT

DATE	TIME
PHONE	EMAIL
SERVICE	DURATION

SUPPLIES

NOTES

CLIENT

DATE	TIME
PHONE	EMAIL
SERVICE	DURATION

SUPPLIES

NOTES

CLIENT

DATE	TIME
PHONE	EMAIL
SERVICE	DURATION

SUPPLIES

NOTES

CLIENT

DATE	TIME
PHONE	EMAIL
SERVICE	DURATION

SUPPLIES

NOTES

CLIENT

DATE	TIME
PHONE	EMAIL
SERVICE	DURATION

SUPPLIES

NOTES

CLIENT

DATE | TIME

PHONE | EMAIL

SERVICE | DURATION

SUPPLIES

NOTES

CLIENT

DATE | TIME

PHONE | EMAIL

SERVICE | DURATION

SUPPLIES

NOTES

CLIENT

DATE | TIME

PHONE | EMAIL

SERVICE | DURATION

SUPPLIES

NOTES

CLIENT

DATE | TIME

PHONE | EMAIL

SERVICE | DURATION

SUPPLIES

NOTES

CLIENT

DATE	TIME
PHONE	EMAIL
SERVICE	DURATION

SUPPLIES

NOTES

CLIENT

DATE	TIME
PHONE	EMAIL
SERVICE	DURATION

SUPPLIES

NOTES

CLIENT

DATE	TIME
PHONE	EMAIL
SERVICE	DURATION

SUPPLIES

NOTES

CLIENT

DATE	TIME
PHONE	EMAIL
SERVICE	DURATION

SUPPLIES

NOTES

CLIENT

DATE	TIME
PHONE	EMAIL
SERVICE	DURATION

SUPPLIES

NOTES

CLIENT

DATE	TIME
PHONE	EMAIL
SERVICE	DURATION

SUPPLIES

NOTES

CLIENT

DATE	TIME
PHONE	EMAIL
SERVICE	DURATION

SUPPLIES

NOTES

CLIENT

DATE	TIME
PHONE	EMAIL
SERVICE	DURATION

SUPPLIES

NOTES

CLIENT

DATE	TIME
PHONE	EMAIL
SERVICE	DURATION

SUPPLIES

NOTES

CLIENT

DATE	TIME
PHONE	EMAIL
SERVICE	DURATION

SUPPLIES

NOTES

CLIENT

DATE	TIME
PHONE	EMAIL
SERVICE	DURATION

SUPPLIES

NOTES

CLIENT

DATE	TIME
PHONE	EMAIL
SERVICE	DURATION

SUPPLIES

NOTES

CLIENT

DATE	TIME
PHONE	EMAIL
SERVICE	DURATION

SUPPLIES

NOTES

CLIENT

DATE	TIME
PHONE	EMAIL
SERVICE	DURATION

SUPPLIES

NOTES

CLIENT

DATE	TIME
PHONE	EMAIL
SERVICE	DURATION

SUPPLIES

NOTES

CLIENT

DATE	TIME
PHONE	EMAIL
SERVICE	DURATION

SUPPLIES

NOTES

CLIENT

DATE	TIME
PHONE	EMAIL
SERVICE	DURATION

SUPPLIES

NOTES

CLIENT

DATE	TIME
PHONE	EMAIL
SERVICE	DURATION

SUPPLIES

NOTES

CLIENT

DATE	TIME
PHONE	EMAIL
SERVICE	DURATION

SUPPLIES

NOTES

CLIENT

DATE	TIME
PHONE	EMAIL
SERVICE	DURATION

SUPPLIES

NOTES

CLIENT

DATE	TIME
PHONE	EMAIL
SERVICE	DURATION

SUPPLIES

NOTES

CLIENT

DATE	TIME
PHONE	EMAIL
SERVICE	DURATION

SUPPLIES

NOTES

CLIENT

DATE | TIME

PHONE | EMAIL

SERVICE | DURATION

SUPPLIES

NOTES

CLIENT

DATE | TIME

PHONE | EMAIL

SERVICE | DURATION

SUPPLIES

NOTES

CLIENT

DATE	TIME
PHONE	EMAIL
SERVICE	DURATION

SUPPLIES

NOTES

CLIENT

DATE	TIME
PHONE	EMAIL
SERVICE	DURATION

SUPPLIES

NOTES

CLIENT

DATE | TIME

PHONE | EMAIL

SERVICE | DURATION

SUPPLIES

NOTES

CLIENT

DATE | TIME

PHONE | EMAIL

SERVICE | DURATION

SUPPLIES

NOTES

CLIENT

DATE	TIME
PHONE	EMAIL
SERVICE	DURATION

SUPPLIES

NOTES

CLIENT

DATE	TIME
PHONE	EMAIL
SERVICE	DURATION

SUPPLIES

NOTES

CLIENT

DATE	TIME
PHONE	EMAIL
SERVICE	DURATION

SUPPLIES

NOTES

CLIENT

DATE	TIME
PHONE	EMAIL
SERVICE	DURATION

SUPPLIES

NOTES

CLIENT

DATE | TIME

PHONE | EMAIL

SERVICE | DURATION

SUPPLIES

NOTES

CLIENT

DATE | TIME

PHONE | EMAIL

SERVICE | DURATION

SUPPLIES

NOTES

CLIENT

DATE	TIME
PHONE	EMAIL
SERVICE	DURATION

SUPPLIES

NOTES

CLIENT

DATE	TIME
PHONE	EMAIL
SERVICE	DURATION

SUPPLIES

NOTES

CLIENT

DATE	TIME
PHONE	EMAIL
SERVICE	DURATION

SUPPLIES

NOTES

CLIENT

DATE	TIME
PHONE	EMAIL
SERVICE	DURATION

SUPPLIES

NOTES

CLIENT

DATE | TIME

PHONE | EMAIL

SERVICE | DURATION

SUPPLIES

NOTES

CLIENT

DATE | TIME

PHONE | EMAIL

SERVICE | DURATION

SUPPLIES

NOTES

CLIENT

DATE	TIME
PHONE	EMAIL
SERVICE	DURATION

SUPPLIES

NOTES

CLIENT

DATE	TIME
PHONE	EMAIL
SERVICE	DURATION

SUPPLIES

NOTES

CLIENT

DATE	TIME
PHONE	EMAIL
SERVICE	DURATION

SUPPLIES

NOTES

CLIENT

DATE	TIME
PHONE	EMAIL
SERVICE	DURATION

SUPPLIES

NOTES

CLIENT

DATE	TIME
PHONE	EMAIL
SERVICE	DURATION

SUPPLIES

NOTES

CLIENT

DATE	TIME
PHONE	EMAIL
SERVICE	DURATION

SUPPLIES

NOTES

CLIENT

DATE	TIME
PHONE	EMAIL
SERVICE	DURATION

SUPPLIES

NOTES

CLIENT

DATE	TIME
PHONE	EMAIL
SERVICE	DURATION

SUPPLIES

NOTES

CLIENT

DATE	TIME
PHONE	EMAIL
SERVICE	DURATION

SUPPLIES

NOTES

CLIENT

DATE	TIME
PHONE	EMAIL
SERVICE	DURATION

SUPPLIES

NOTES

CLIENT

DATE	TIME
PHONE	EMAIL
SERVICE	DURATION

SUPPLIES

NOTES

CLIENT

DATE	TIME
PHONE	EMAIL
SERVICE	DURATION

SUPPLIES

NOTES

CLIENT

DATE	TIME
PHONE	EMAIL
SERVICE	DURATION

SUPPLIES

NOTES

CLIENT

DATE	TIME
PHONE	EMAIL
SERVICE	DURATION

SUPPLIES

NOTES

CLIENT

DATE	TIME
PHONE	EMAIL
SERVICE	DURATION

SUPPLIES

NOTES

CLIENT

DATE	TIME
PHONE	EMAIL
SERVICE	DURATION

SUPPLIES

NOTES

CLIENT

DATE	TIME
PHONE	EMAIL
SERVICE	DURATION

SUPPLIES

NOTES

CLIENT

DATE	TIME
PHONE	EMAIL
SERVICE	DURATION

SUPPLIES

NOTES

CLIENT

DATE	TIME
PHONE	EMAIL
SERVICE	DURATION

SUPPLIES

NOTES

CLIENT

DATE	TIME
PHONE	EMAIL
SERVICE	DURATION

SUPPLIES

NOTES

CLIENT

DATE	TIME
PHONE	EMAIL
SERVICE	DURATION

SUPPLIES

NOTES

CLIENT

DATE	TIME
PHONE	EMAIL
SERVICE	DURATION

SUPPLIES

NOTES

CLIENT

DATE	TIME
PHONE	EMAIL
SERVICE	DURATION

SUPPLIES

NOTES

CLIENT

DATE	TIME
PHONE	EMAIL
SERVICE	DURATION

SUPPLIES

NOTES

CLIENT

DATE	TIME
PHONE	EMAIL
SERVICE	DURATION

SUPPLIES

NOTES

CLIENT

DATE	TIME
PHONE	EMAIL
SERVICE	DURATION

SUPPLIES

NOTES

CLIENT

DATE	TIME
PHONE	EMAIL
SERVICE	DURATION

SUPPLIES

NOTES

CLIENT

DATE	TIME
PHONE	EMAIL
SERVICE	DURATION

SUPPLIES

NOTES

CLIENT

DATE | TIME

PHONE | EMAIL

SERVICE | DURATION

SUPPLIES

NOTES

CLIENT

DATE | TIME

PHONE | EMAIL

SERVICE | DURATION

SUPPLIES

NOTES

CLIENT

DATE	TIME
PHONE	EMAIL
SERVICE	DURATION

SUPPLIES

NOTES

CLIENT

DATE	TIME
PHONE	EMAIL
SERVICE	DURATION

SUPPLIES

NOTES

CLIENT

DATE	TIME
PHONE	EMAIL
SERVICE	DURATION

SUPPLIES

NOTES

CLIENT

DATE	TIME
PHONE	EMAIL
SERVICE	DURATION

SUPPLIES

NOTES

CLIENT

DATE	TIME
PHONE	EMAIL
SERVICE	DURATION

SUPPLIES

NOTES

CLIENT

DATE	TIME
PHONE	EMAIL
SERVICE	DURATION

SUPPLIES

NOTES

CLIENT

DATE	TIME
PHONE	EMAIL
SERVICE	DURATION

SUPPLIES

NOTES

CLIENT

DATE	TIME
PHONE	EMAIL
SERVICE	DURATION

SUPPLIES

NOTES

CLIENT

DATE	TIME
PHONE	EMAIL
SERVICE	DURATION

SUPPLIES

NOTES

CLIENT

DATE	TIME
PHONE	EMAIL
SERVICE	DURATION

SUPPLIES

NOTES

CLIENT

DATE | TIME
PHONE | EMAIL
SERVICE | DURATION

SUPPLIES

NOTES

CLIENT

DATE | TIME
PHONE | EMAIL
SERVICE | DURATION

SUPPLIES

NOTES

CLIENT

DATE	TIME
PHONE	EMAIL
SERVICE	DURATION

SUPPLIES

NOTES

CLIENT

DATE	TIME
PHONE	EMAIL
SERVICE	DURATION

SUPPLIES

NOTES

CLIENT

DATE	TIME
PHONE	EMAIL
SERVICE	DURATION

SUPPLIES

NOTES

CLIENT

DATE	TIME
PHONE	EMAIL
SERVICE	DURATION

SUPPLIES

NOTES

CLIENT

DATE | TIME

PHONE | EMAIL

SERVICE | DURATION

SUPPLIES

NOTES

CLIENT

DATE | TIME

PHONE | EMAIL

SERVICE | DURATION

SUPPLIES

NOTES

CLIENT

DATE	TIME
PHONE	EMAIL
SERVICE	DURATION

SUPPLIES

NOTES

CLIENT

DATE	TIME
PHONE	EMAIL
SERVICE	DURATION

SUPPLIES

NOTES

CLIENT

DATE	TIME
PHONE	EMAIL
SERVICE	DURATION

SUPPLIES

NOTES

CLIENT

DATE	TIME
PHONE	EMAIL
SERVICE	DURATION

SUPPLIES

NOTES

www.ingramcontent.com/pod-product-compliance
Lightning Source LLC
Chambersburg PA
CBHW070847250726
48662CB00003B/1400